Epilepsy in Elderly People

Raymond Tallis, FRCP
Professor of Geriatric Medicine
University of Manchester Department of Geriatric Medicine, and Physician in Health Care of the Elderly
Salford Royal Hospitals Trust

MARTIN DUNITZ

First published in the United Kingdom
in 1995 by

Martin Dunitz Ltd
The Livery House
7–9 Pratt Street
London NW1 0AE

A CIP record for this book is available from the British Library.

ISBN 1-85317-244-8
Printed and bound in Spain by Cayfosa

Contents

Preface – Epilepsy in old age is important and different

Until recently, elderly-onset seizures have been comparatively neglected and a book devoted specifically to epilepsy in elderly people might have been thought unnecessary. Many doctors still believe that epilepsy only rarely begins in old age.[1] Some mistakenly think that seizures in the elderly are less important than those that affect younger people. Others imagine that what we know of epilepsy in the general adult population may be applied directly to elderly people. All of these assumptions are incorrect.

Seizures in old age are important

First and foremost, there is the actual experience of the seizure; there is no need to emphasize the unpleasantness of this for the patient. In older people, post-ictal states are often prolonged beyond the traditional 24 hours, sometimes persisting as long as a week.[2,3] Todd's phenomena are also more common, especially post-ictal hemiparesis. Although no adequate prospective studies have been undertaken, it might be anticipated that fits in the elderly more often lead to injury, especially as osteoporotic bones in older people are more liable to fracture.

Fits may have wider and more chronic consequences. Several studies (reviewed recently by Downton[4]) have confirmed how a fall may mark a watershed in an older person's life, after which there is a sharp decline in functional independence. In some instances this will be due to the disease that underlies the fall, but in many more cases it will be due to a loss of confidence. The well-known 3 Fs (*Fear of Further Falls*) that may cause an elderly person to become semi-electively housebound must surely have its analogue in *Fear of Further Fits.* The frightening experience of a fit may seem like a harbinger of death. This fear may be greater in elderly people who may have known a contemporary who has died after 'a funny turn' or who may have distant memories of a childhood when epilepsy was stigmatized, poorly controlled, very much an affair of the street or the institution and often, partly due to the adverse effects of toxic but useless drugs, associated with severe chronic impairment of mental function.

The impact of seizures will also include their adverse effect on the attitudes of others, including friends, relatives and carers, to the patient, resulting in:

- Decreased activity
- More exclusion from decision making processes
- More susceptibility to interference in their affairs by others
- Less grandparental involvement in child rearing

In summary, marginalization, disempowerment and a shrinkage of life-space.

So, although the diagnosis of seizures will not have the effects on employment and education that it may have in a younger person, the impact on interpersonal relations may be no less important. Elderly people may be more dependent on motorized transport for mobility; and, if the individual who has the fit is the only licence holder, the consequent exclusion from driving may mean that *two* people are housebound.

Seizures in old age are different

The following summarizes some of the ways in which seizures may be expected to be different in older people and therefore worthy of separate consideration.

Seizures in old age are different	
Presentation	The history is frequently inadequate and the diagnosis – especially distinguishing seizures from cardiovascular causes of episodic loss of consciousness – particularly difficult
Aetiology	Seizures will be more often symptomatic and more likely due to underlying focal cerebral lesions, in particular cerebrovascular disease
Co–morbidity	Concurrent pathology unrelated to the seizures is common and the patient will frequently be on medication other than anti-epileptic drugs (AEDs)
Functional consequences	As elderly patients may already be close to the threshold of functional failure, fits and the adverse effects of their treatment may be more likely to cause loss of confidence and even of independence
Clinical pharmacology	The kinetics and dynamics of AEDs may be altered, partly due to age but, more importantly, to co-morbidity and concurrent medication

Introduction

Epileptic seizures are the clinical manifestations of hyperexcitability of the neurones in the cerebral hemispheres. The electrical activity is spontaneous and independent of the normal discharges that are associated with motor activity and sensory processing. It originates in the cerebral cortex and is both excessive in quantity and excessively synchronized.

It is important to distinguish between an epileptic seizure and epilepsy:

An epileptic seizure	is an intermittent, stereotyped disturbance of consciousness, motor function, sensation, perception, emotion, or behaviour that clinically appears to be due to inappropriate, excessive cortical neuronal activity
Epilepsy	is a propensity to suffer from recurrent, usually unprovoked seizures

It follows that a diagnosis of epilepsy cannot strictly be made on the basis of a single seizure, especially if the seizure seems to have a provoking cause. For epidemiological purposes 'epilepsy' is defined as two or more unprovoked seizures. The distinction, however, is not as sharp as is sometimes implied; in old age at least, the majority of individuals who present with a single seizure will go on to have further seizures.[5-7]

Classification of seizures and epilepsy

There are many reasons for trying to classify seizures and types of epileptic syndromes. In the individual patient, this may:

- Suggest an underlying cause or condition
- Point to the prognosis (including the prognosis for control)
- Guide the choice of anti-convulsants

Classification may also give researchers clues as to the kinds of underlying mechanisms that should be sought; for example, unprovoked primarily generalized seizures are more likely to have a genetic basis, while partial seizures are more likely to result from acquired focal cerebral damage.

Unfortunately, this worthy aim has generated extremely complex schemes of classification that non-experts find difficult to use. However, many of the types of seizures described in the standard classifications are not found in elderly-onset cases. Moreover, as most seizures in old age respond to broad spectrum anti-epileptic drugs (AEDs), classification is not usually necessary to guide treatment. Table 1 provides a classification for seizures occurring in the elderly.

The classification of **epileptic syndromes**, as opposed to types of seizures, is even more complex, being based on a

Partial seizures: focal onset

Simple: consciousness unimpaired throughout

With motor symptoms:
- focal motor with or without march
- versive
- postural
- vocalization

With somatosensory or special-sensory symptoms:
- somatosensory
- visual
- auditory
- olfactory
- gustatory
- vertiginous

With autonomic symptoms or signs:
- epigastric sensations
- pallor
- sweating
- flushing
- piloerection
- pupillary dilation

With disturbances of higher cerebral function:
- dysphasic
- dysmnestic
- cognitive
- affective

Illusions (e.g. macropsia)

Structured hallucinations (e.g. music, scenes)

cont.

Partial seizures: focal onset

Complex: consciousness impaired at some point

Beginning as simple partial seizures and progressing to complex seizures

Consciousness impaired from the outset:
- impairment of consciousness only
- impairment of consciousness with automatism

Partial seizures becoming secondarily generalized (with convulsive manifestations)

Generalized seizures: onset is generalized

- Myoclonic seizures
- Clonic seizures
- Tonic seizures
- Tonic-clonic seizures
- Atonic seizures

Note: brief absences occurring in older people are most often due to complex partial seizures (they used to be called 'temporal lobe absences'). They are not 'petit mal' – you have to be 'petit' to have 'petit mal'!

Table 1
Classification of seizures occurring in elderly people (modified from reference 8).

bewildering combination of clinical manifestations of seizures, presumed aetiologies, age of onset and electroencephalographic findings.[9] Again, most of the syndromes are not found in old age and so these complex classification schemes are not relevant.

Epidemiology of epilepsy and epileptic seizures

The belief that elderly-onset seizures are uncommon has no foundation in the literature. Hauser and Kurland[10] reported a rise in the prevalence of epilepsy above the age of 50 and an even steeper rise in incidence – from 12 per 100 000 in the 40–59 year age group to 82 per 100 000 in those over 60. These authors confirmed this rise in more recent studies,[11,12] and Luhdorf[13] reported a similar incidence of 77 per 100 000.

These findings have also been confirmed by studies based in primary care. The United Kingdom National General Practice Study of Epilepsy and Epileptic Seizures, a prospective community-based study, found that 24% of new cases of definite epilepsy were in subjects over the age of 60.[5] A study of a primary care database covering 82 practices and nearly 370 000 subjects, 62 000 of whom were over the age of 60, revealed a continuing rise in the incidence of seizures in old age:[14] the incidence for the overall population was 69 per 100 000, but in the 65–69 age group it was 87, in the 70–79 group it was 147, and in the 80–89 group it was 159 per 100 000. Over a third of all incident cases placed on AEDs were over the age of 60. Analysis of an expanded primary care database of over 3 million subjects has generated very similar findings (Tallis et al, in preparation).

The high incidence is observed for both definite epilepsy and single seizures. In a study by Loiseau,[15] the annual incidence for all seizures (single and recurrent) was 127 per 100 000 in subjects over 60, and the over-60s accounted for 28% of cases of confirmed epilepsy (two or more unprovoked seizures) and 52% of acute symptomatic seizures. The Rochester Minnesota survey[12] also found that both single unprovoked seizures and definite epilepsy increased sharply with age.

The dramatic rise of the incidence of seizures with age is illustrated in Figure 1. In view of the predicted rise in the elderly population (Figure 2), a parallel rise in the number of cases of elderly-onset seizures may be anticipated.

The classification of seizures in old age in epidemiological studies is less certain. Large, population-based studies do not have full electrophysiological evaluation, which is important because seizures that appear clinically to be primarily generalized may actually be focal in origin (and symptomatic), though generalization occurs too rapidly to be noted by an observer.

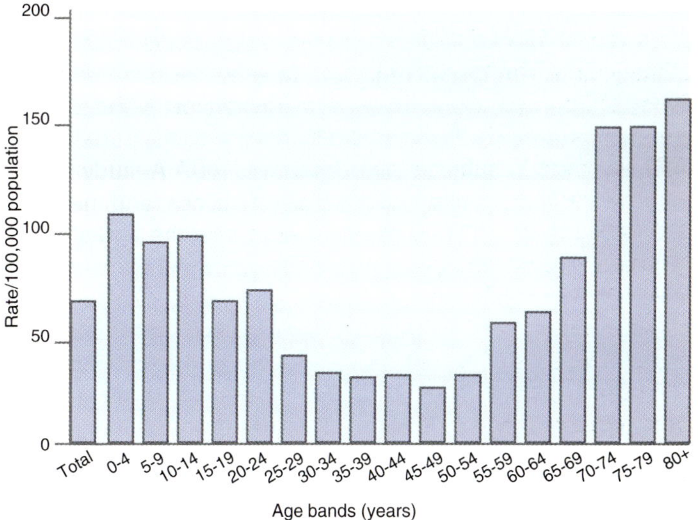

Figure 1

The age-related incidence of seizures (reproduced with permission from Tallis et al[14]).

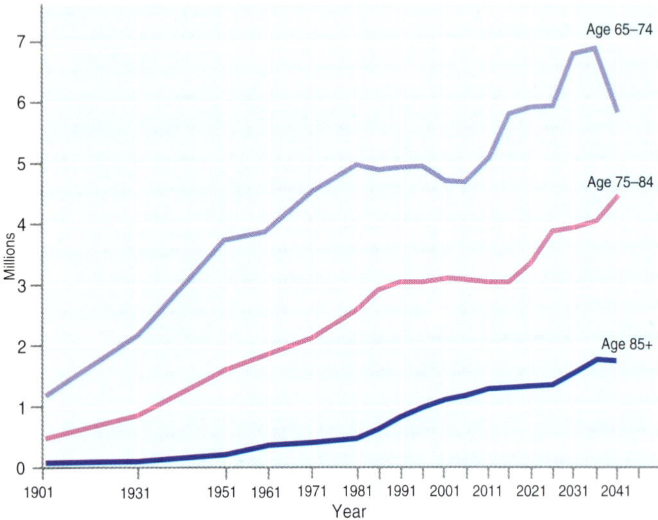

Figure 2

Population projections (reproduced with kind permission from Laing W, Hall M. Agenda for health 1991 – The challenges of ageing. London: Association of the British Pharmaceutical Industry, 1991).

Studies in which investigation has been adequate to ensure classification are often derived from atypical populations attending neuromedical centres. Current evidence suggests that at least 75% of elderly-onset seizures are focal or focal in origin.[5] The real figure may be higher as it seems unlikely that primary generalized seizures occur spontaneously for the first time in old age. An individual with an idiopathic lowered seizure threshold would have expressed this earlier in life.

Aetiology

Epilepsy, like incontinence, is not a diagnosis but a symptom. The majority of seizures in old age are secondary, though a definite cause is not always established. The proportions attributed to different causes must be regarded as provisional until results are available from large population-based studies in which all cases have been adequately investigated.

Cerebrovascular disease

The commonest cause of elderly onset seizures is cerebrovascular disease, which accounts for 30–50% of cases in different series.[5,15–17] It accounts for an even higher proportion – nearly 75%[5] – of those cases in which a definite cause is found. There are several ways in which seizures and cerebrovascular disease may be connected:

Seizures may be associated with overt stroke
- early
- late

Patients with late-onset seizures may have occult cerebrovascular disease
- concurrent CT scan finding
- subsequent development of stroke

About 4% of stroke patients have early seizures[18] and seizures occur within five years of an ischaemic stroke in about 10% of cases (Sandercock, personal communication of unpublished data from the Oxford Community Stroke Project). Haemorrhagic stroke is associated with a higher incidence of seizures.[19]

The more carefully cerebrovascular disease is sought in late-onset epileptic patients, the more frequently it is identified.[20] This observation may have to be treated with some caution – the presence of areas of ischaemia on a CT scan may not mean that these are the cause of the seizures.

Finally, seizures may be the first manifestation of hitherto silent cerebrovascular disease: there is an excess of previous seizures in patients admitted to hospital with an acute stroke compared with controls, suggesting that clinically undetectable cerebrovascular disease may present with seizures and that an otherwise unexplained elderly onset seizure may warn of future stroke.[21] *The practical significance of this is that any elderly patient with unexplained seizures should be fully screened for cardiovascular risk factors and treatment with low dose aspirin or other preventative measures should be instituted where appropriate.*

The strong relationship between age and the incidence and prevalence of cerebrovascular disease – as reflected in the almost exponential relationship between age and first-ever stroke (Figure 3) – underlines the importance of this cause of elderly-onset seizures.

Cerebral tumours

Between 5% and 15% of cases of elderly onset seizures are associated with cerebral tumours.[5,16,17] In one large study from south west France,[15] 22% of cases of recurrent unprovoked seizures were associated with cerebral tumours, but this is exceptional. Most tumours are either metastatic or

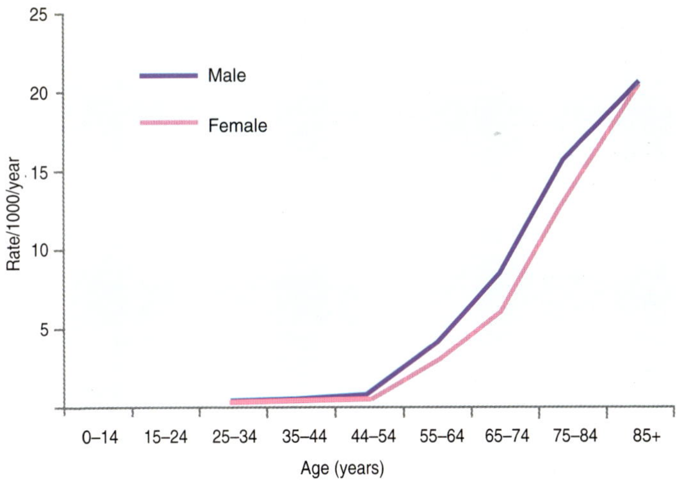

Figure 3
Age-related incidence of stroke (n=675) in the Oxfordshire Community Stroke Project (reproduced with kind permission from Bamford, Sandercock, Dennis et al. A prospective study of acute cerebrovascular disease in the community. Journal of Neurology, Neurosurgery and Psychiatry 1988; ***51****:1373 – 80).*

(inoperable) gliomas, with few meningiomas, although these are diagnosed from time to time (Figure 4). However, until an adequately documented, adequately investigated and sufficiently large population-based study has been carried out, the proportion of very late onset epilepsy that is due to treatable and non-treatable tumours cannot be ascertained. At any rate, the proportion of seizures due to tumours without any pointers to the underlying cause – such as progressive neurological signs or features suggestive of raised intracranial pressure – will be quite small.

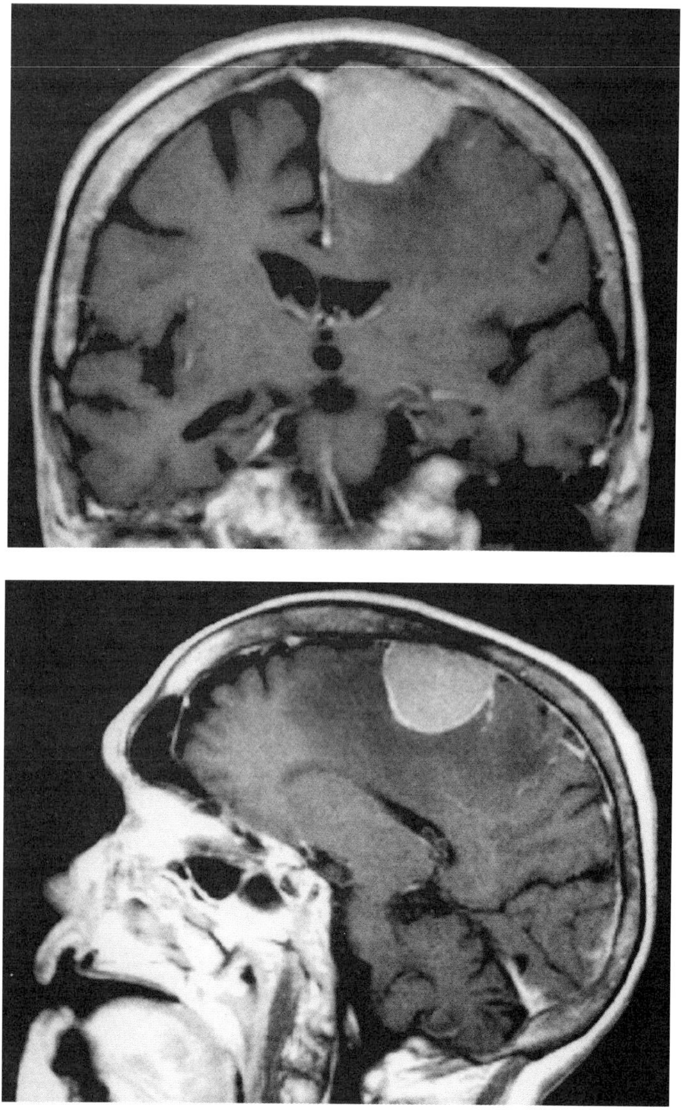

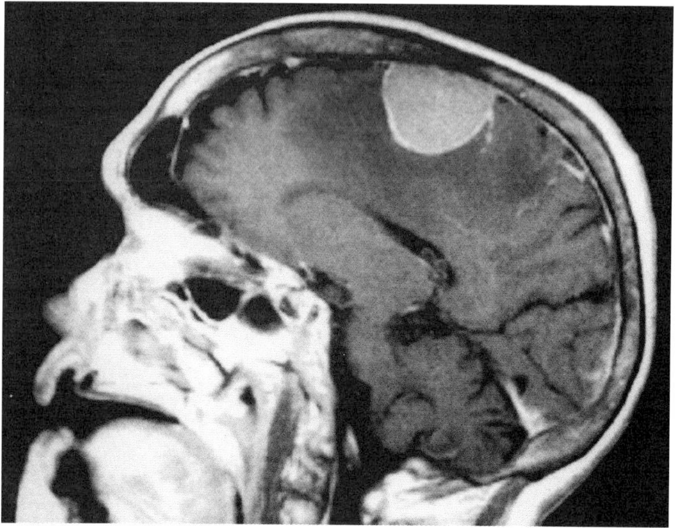

Figure 4
MRI scan showing a meningioma in an 82-year-old female who presented with seizures commencing 2 years earlier (reproduced with kind permission of the Department of Magnetic Resonance Imaging, Salford Royal Hospitals Trust).

Non-vascular dementia

It is unclear whether non-vascular dementias such as Alzheimer's disease cause seizures as some, such as Mcareavy et al,[22] have suggested. There have been no sufficiently large studies in which 'gold standard' diagnostic criteria have been used to rule out either the alternative diagnosis of multi-infarct dementia or mixed vascular and non-vascular dementia.

Toxic and metabolic causes

These include:

- Pyrexia
- Hypoglycaemia
- Electrolyte disturbances (including water overload)
- Hypoxia with or without respiratory failure
- Severe myxoedema
- Hepatic failure
- Renal failure
- Drugs and drug withdrawal
- Alcohol and alcohol withdrawal

Recent studies, such as that by Luhdorf et al,[16] have underlined the importance of toxic and metabolic causes of seizures in old age. Alcohol is important at any age.[23,24] Pyrexia and other acute conditions may precipitate seizures in older people[15] and pneumonia, which may be more likely to cause hypoxia in the biologically aged,[25] may predispose to seizures or precipitate them in an individual who has otherwise well-controlled epilepsy. Many drugs cause confusion and convulsions.[26,27] Drug-induced seizures are particularly likely when blood levels are high; this is often the case in patients with impaired drug handling – a category which will include many elderly people. Drugs suspected of being epileptogenic are listed in Table 2.

Drugs that may cause seizures	
Antibiotics	Benzylpenicillin Oxacillin Carbenicillin Isoniazid Cycloserine
Hormones	Insulin Oral hypoglycaemics Prednisone
Local anaesthetics/anti-arrhythmics	Lignocaine Procaine Disopyramide Anticholinergics in overdose
Psychotropic drugs	Chlorpromazine Other phenothiazines Tricyclic antidepressants Lithium
Analeptic drugs	Aminophylline Doxapram
Anaesthetic agents	Ether Methohexitone Ketamine Halothane Althesin
Radiographic contrast media	Meglumine Metrizamide (very rare)
Withdrawal fits	Benzodiazepines Alcohol

Table 2
Drugs that may cause seizures (after Chadwick[26]).

Diagnosis and investigation

The diagnostic task when a patient presents with suspected seizures is complex (Figure 5). There are three main tools that can be used to answer the questions posed in Figure 5:

1. The most powerful tool is a detailed history. For obvious reasons, the history from the patient may be unsatisfactory and eye witness reports must be sought. This may be difficult in a patient who lives alone and who has simply been 'found on the floor'. Even evidence from people – neighbours, ambulance drivers, casualty staff – who did not see the event itself but observed the patient's post-event state may be helpful. In the case of an elderly person living alone, this may be the only source of useful history.

2. The next most powerful tool is a wide-ranging, open-minded, physical examination.

3. The third most powerful tool is time. It is better to wait and see than to initiate inappropriate treatment.

Are the events seizures?

In the case of a classical generalized or partial seizure, the diagnosis can be readily made on the basis of the history. Unfortunately, fits may be difficult to differentiate from a variety of non-epileptic paroxysmal events that also occur in elderly people, such as:

- Syncope
- Hypoglycaemia
- Transient ischaemic attacks
- Recurrent paroxysmal behavioural disturbances secondary to organic brain disease
- Drop attacks and other non-epileptic causes of falls
- Transient global amnesia
- Psychogenic attacks
  - panic attacks
  - hyperventilation
  - pseudo-seizures

Some of these may be relatively easily ruled out, while others are more difficult to differentiate from seizures:

1. **Hypoglycaemia** is rare in a patient not on hypoglycaemic medication. Where it does occur, however, it may not in an elderly person be associated with characteristic autonomic features.[28] Nocturnal hypoglycaemia due to longer-acting oral hypoglycaemics such as chlorpropamide and glibenclamide may occasionally cause fits and present as early morning confusion and post-ictal headache.

2. **Transient ischaemic attacks** do not typically cause disturbance of consciousness. They tend to have negative features, such as weakness and numbness, whereas focal seizures have positive features such as twitching and tingling or lancinating sensations.[29]

3. **Recurrent paroxysmal behavioural disturbances** are seen in dementias, in particular multi-infarct states. They may be confused with complex partial seizures (or vice versa – see below). Unlike the latter, they tend to have a predictable diurnal pattern, occurring as darkness falls – the so-called 'sundowner effect'.[30]

4. **Drop attacks** typically occur in middle age, are associated with immediate (rather embarrassed) recovery, and do not cause loss of consciousness: "my legs just gave way, doctor". They tend to occur in a cluster and spontaneously remit. Other causes of recurrent falls may be inappropriately attributed to seizures. However, the reverse error is more likely – fits may not be considered when the only available history is that the patient is repeatedly being found on the floor.

5. **Transient global amnesia** may be confused with complex partial seizures causing temporal lobe dysfunction and consequent memory disturbance. However, it is less common, has characteristic features (anguished dis-

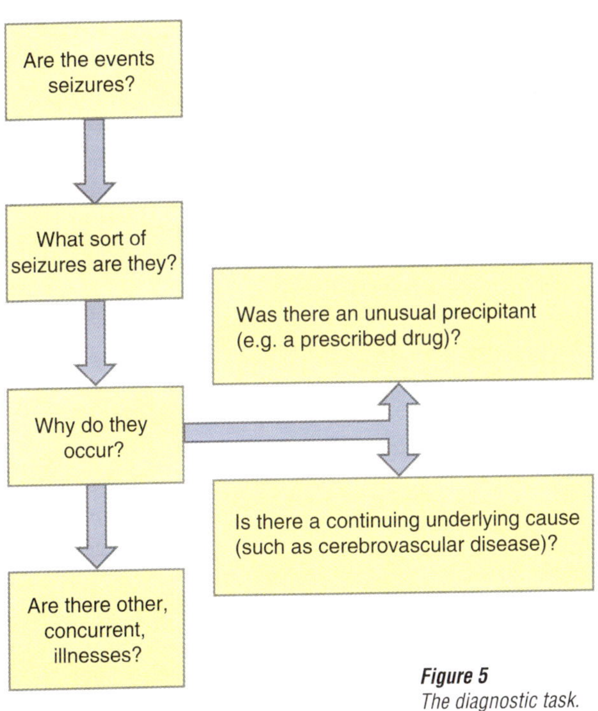

Figure 5
The diagnostic task.

orientation and repeated asking of the same questions), typically lasts for 24 hours and does not usually recur.[31]

6. It is unusual for **psychogenic attacks** to occur for the first time in old age and there are typically other features of functional psychiatric illness and precipitating factors such as bereavement. The difference between epileptic seizures and pseudo-seizures is explained in more detail on page 26 of Appleton et al.[32]

7. The most difficult differential diagnosis is **syncope**. Even when there is a reasonably good history, the features that characteristically differentiate fits from faints may not be as decisive as in younger adults, as is shown in Table 3.

Differentiating fits from faints may be even more difficult when there are coexistent conditions predisposing to both syncope and seizures. Moreover, it is well known that transient cerebral anoxia, as for example in vagal hypersensitivity – now recognized to be much more common than hitherto realized [33] – may itself cause convulsions. Recurrent cardiac arrhythmias are particularly important: in one series of patients referred to a neurological department with a diagnosis of epilepsy, 20% were found to have cardiac arrhythmias that caused or significantly contributed to their symptoms.[34] The situation may be particularly confusing, as complex partial seizures affecting the temporal lobes may present with autonomic features.

It may, therefore, prove impossible to determine whether transient cerebral symptoms are cardiac or cerebral in origin. Even ambulatory 24-hour ECG, with or without other cardiovascular tests, and prolonged EEG monitoring may not permit a confident diagnosis. Non-specific abnormalities on an EEG, or cardiac arrythmias recorded on a 24 hour tape but unrelated to the symptoms, may add to the confusion. Head-up tilt for up to 45 minutes with or without carotid sinus massage may induce bradycardia and/or hypotension and thus help differentiate syncope from epilepsy.[35]

Features	Usual distinction		Modifications in older patients
	Faints	**Fits**	
Posture	Usually occur in the upright position	Not position-dependent	Faints in older people are not position-dependent because they are often due to significant, position-independent, pathology
Onset	Gradual	Sudden	Loss of consciousness may be quite abrupt in syncope in an older person; complex partial seizures may have a gradual onset
Injury	Rare	More common	A syncopal attack may be associated with significant soft tissue or bony injury in an older person
Incontinence	Rare	Common	An individual prone to incontinence may be wet during a faint; partial seizures will not usually be associated with incontinence
Recovery	Rapid	Slow	A fit may take the form of a brief ('temporal lobe') absence; a faint associated with a serious arrhythmia may be prolonged
Post-event confusion	Little	Marked	A prolonged hypoxic episode due to a faint may be associated with prolonged post-event confusion
Frequency	Usually infrequent with a clear precipitating cause	May be frequent and usually without precipitating cause	Faints associated with cardiac arrythmias, low cardiac output, postural hypotension or carotid sinus sensitivity may be very frequent

Table 3
The differences between faints and fits: problems in older patients.

Some genuinely epileptic events may not be appreciated for what they are (Table 4).

Complex partial seizures, with or without automatisms, may be labelled as non-specific confusional states or even, where there are affective[37] or cognitive features or hallucinations, as manifestations of functional psychiatric illnesses. Patients with non-convulsive epileptic status may present with acute behavioural changes – withdrawal, mutism, delusional ideas, paranoia, vivid hallucinations and fugue states.[38] Fluctuating mental impairment may easily be attributed to other causes of recurrent confusional states or even misread as part of a dementing process.[39,40] Alternatively, there may be abrupt loss of consciousness without tonic/clonic movements – so-called akinetic seizures.[3]

Todd's paresis after a fit may be misdiagnosed as stroke; indeed, in one series this was the commonest non-stroke cause of referral to a stroke unit.[41] This is particularly likely where fits occur against a background of known cerebrovascular disease, and a recurrence of stroke may be incorrectly diagnosed.[42]

Table 4
Seizures that may be confused with other conditions.

Epileptic event	Possible misdiagnosis
Epilepsia partialis continua (partial motor status)	Extra-pyramidal movement disorder
Sensory epilepsy	Transient ischaemic attack
Complex partial seizures	Organic or functional psychosis
Akinetic seizures	Drop attacks/hysteria
Epileptic vertigo[36] (due to temporal lobe attacks)	Brain stem/vestibular disease/non-specific dizziness
Todd's palsy	Stroke/transient ischaemic attack
Any kind of seizures	'Falls'

In the face of such difficulties, the clinician's primary duty is to acknowledge uncertainty where it exists and, if uncertainty remains after a careful history (including a history of medication and alcohol consumption) has been obtained and a comprehensive examination (including testing for postural hypotension) and appropriate investigations carried out, simply to wait and see. A 'therapeutic trial' of anti-convulsants as a diagnostic test is not recommended: it will rarely produce a clear answer and will add the burden of possibly unnecessary drug treatment to the patient's troubles.

General investigations

The following general investigations should be carried out:

- Full blood count
- ESR
- Urea and electrolytes
- Blood glucose
- Chest X-ray
- Electrocardiogram

Biochemical tests should include an estimate of gamma glutamyl transferase as a marker of recent alcohol consumption and the threshold for carrying out thyroid function tests should be low, as myxoedema (which is occasionally associated with seizures) is common in older people and may present atypically. Other investigations, such as serological testing for syphilis, will be influenced by the history and examination.

The place of special investigations

Lumbar puncture is rarely indicated, except when a fit occurs in the context of an acute illness suggestive of meningitis or when chronic neurological infection is possible. Skull X-ray is rarely informative. EEG and specialized neuro-imaging have their place, although their role is often misunderstood.

Electroencephalography (EEG)

Excessive reliance upon an EEG to make or refute a diagnosis of epilepsy is potentially dangerous at any age. A routine EEG may support the diagnosis of epilepsy, especially if clear-cut paroxysmal discharges are observed (Figure 6). The absence of such activity on a routine recording does not, however, rule out the diagnosis; after all, most recordings last for only 20 minutes

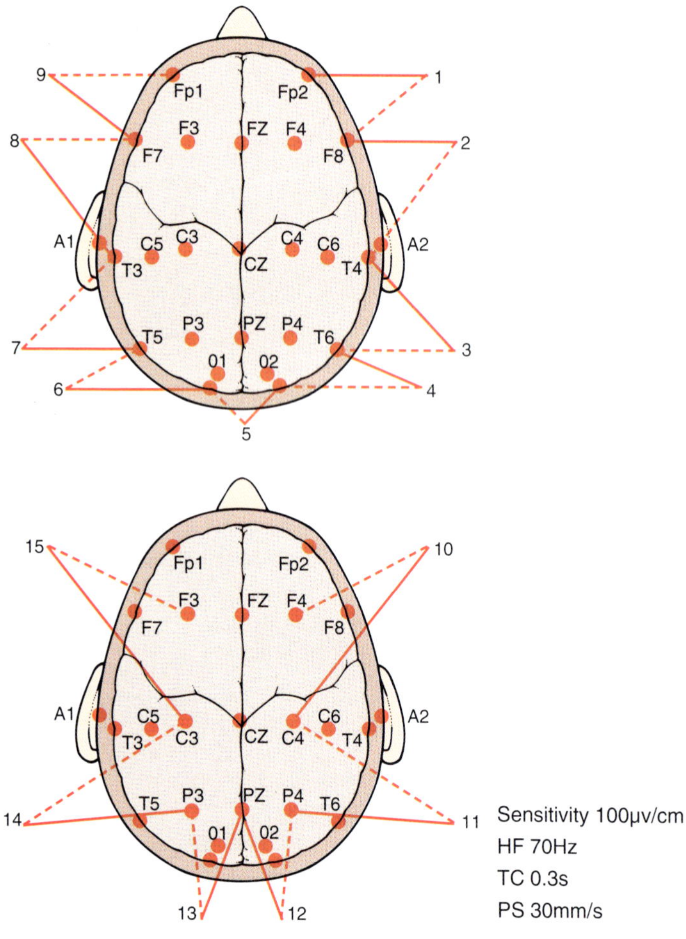

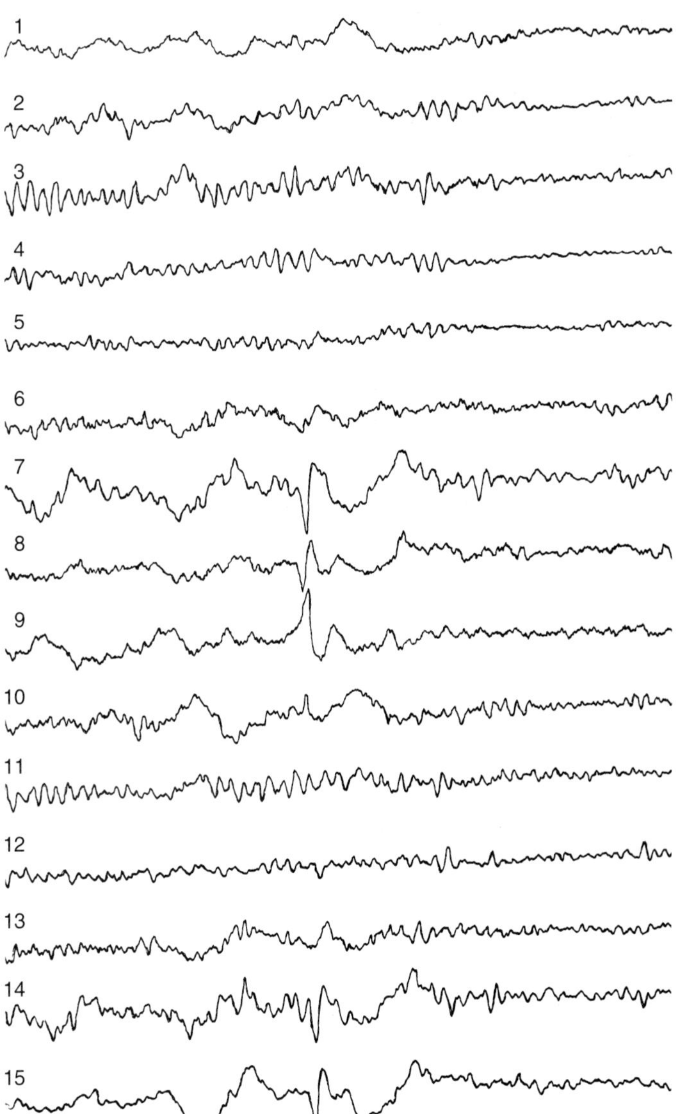

Figure 6
EEG in a patient with elderly-onset seizures showing left temporo-parietal sharp waves (above). (Record reproduced with kind permission of the Department of Clinical Neurophysiology, Salford Royal Hospitals Trust.)

and ictal or pathognomonic inter-ictal activity occurs only intermittently. The range of 'normal' increases with age, so that discriminating 'normal' from 'abnormal' becomes more difficult in an elderly patient, and non-specific abnormalities are common.[43] Thus, while the EEG may provide useful supporting evidence for the diagnosis of epilepsy, it should not overrule the clinical diagnosis nor provide its sole basis. Prolonged (24 hour) EEG recording or telemetry with recording of symptoms may be helpful, although this should take place only on expert advice because of the expense involved.

In elderly people, as in any other age group, EEG alone cannot determine the need for treatment in a newly diagnosed case, establish the adequacy of treatment, or predict the safety of discontinuing therapy. In those fits where there is an inadequate history or where the focal phase is too brief to be observed clinically, the EEG may suggest a focal origin for the first time and guide further investigation. Non-epileptogenic focal abnormal activity, such as a focal slow wave, may raise the suspicion of a progressive lesion, thereby justifying further investigations with neuro-imaging. Ictal or profuse inter-ictal discharges may be particularly useful in diagnosing non-convulsive status or epilepsy presenting with recurrent behavioural disturbance or other neuropsychiatric manifestations.

Computerized tomography (CT)

The older the age of the patient at presentation with epilepsy, the greater the chance of a positive CT scan: as many as 60% of very late onset epilepsy patients may show a structural lesion.[44] This, however, would be an argument for routine scanning only if identification of such lesions influenced management[45] – as in the case of a space-occupying lesion amenable to neurosurgical removal. However, in only a minority of elderly patients with late-onset seizures is a neoplasm or subdural haematoma the cause, and in only a small proportion of cases with tumours would neurosurgical intervention be appropriate. Even where a benign tumour such as a meningioma is diagnosed, neurosurgical treatment may not be indicated:[46] some

Table 5
Indications for computerized tomography in elderly-onset seizures.

STRONG
Unexplained focal neurological signs
Progressive or new neurological symptoms, especially those of raised intracranial pressure
Progressive or new neurological signs
Poor control of fits not attributable to poor compliance with anti-epileptic drugs or continued exposure to precipitants such as alcohol

LESS STRONG
Clear cut, stereotyped focal fits
Persistent marked slow-wave abnormality on the EEG

meningiomas in old age may be relatively inert and craniotomy is often tolerated poorly by elderly patients. Nevertheless, it may be useful to have a definitive diagnosis, even though treatment for the underlying condition may not be available or considered inappropriate. Arguable indications for CT scanning are shown in Table 5.

Magnetic resonance imaging (MRI)

MRI has been assessed in patients with seizures in whom there was no clear cause and CT scans have been normal. In some such cases, MRI has given diagnostically helpful information, confirming that it is a powerful and sensitive diagnostic tool; whether the information obtained using MRI would often alter management in elderly-onset epilepsy remains to be seen.[47]

Management

Aspects of the management of epilepsy in elderly patients are summarized in Figure 7.

Reassurance

In view of what has been said at the outset about older people's views of seizures (see pages 1–2), reassurance is of paramount importance:

- In the vast majority of cases, fits *do not* indicate serious brain damage
- Fits *do not* imply psychiatric disease or dementia
- Fits *can* be controlled by medication
- The medication itself *does not* cause cumulative damage (a frequent worry with elderly people)

The nature of seizures should be explained.

Information

Patients may want to know whether fits are brought on by any particular activity and whether, for this reason, they should lead restricted lives. The advice in this age group is the same as that given to any patient: avoid only those activities that would

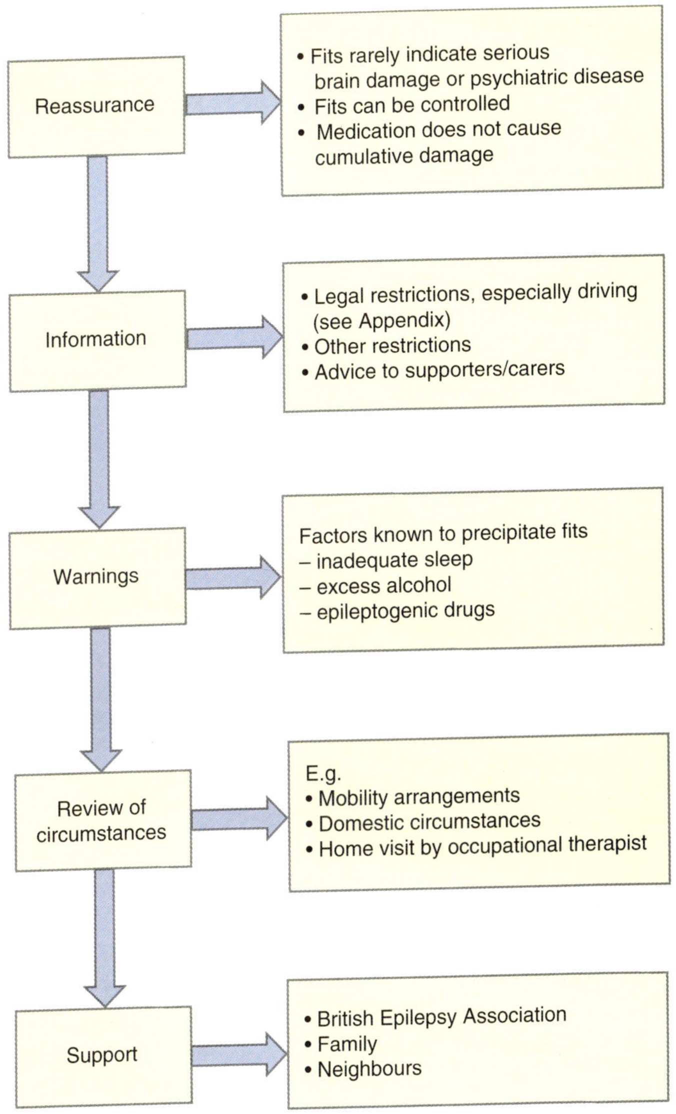

Figure 7
Aspects of the management of epilepsy in elderly people.

mean immediate danger if a fit occurred. This may be less restrictive in an older person than in a younger person.

One such restriction includes **driving**. The regulations regarding driving and epilepsy have recently been revised and are detailed in the Appendix (page 52). Patients should be informed of the regulations and of their responsibility to notify the DVLA, which decides on restrictions. Patients should not drive in the interim.

Warnings

Factors that are known to precipitate fits, such as inadequate sleep or excess alcohol, should be avoided. The patient should be warned that alcohol will increase the side-effects of medication and that other drugs may have a convulsant effect or may interact with AEDs. Patients should remind their doctors that they have epilepsy when they are seen about other conditions for which they may receive prescriptions. Existing medication should be reviewed and drugs known to be potentially epileptogenic or liable to interfere with AEDs should be withdrawn if possible.

Review of circumstances

As so often in old age medicine, management is multi-disciplinary. A fit may cause severe loss of confidence and, in individuals who already have locomotor or other disabilities, this may lead not only to voluntary restriction of activities and a shrinkage of 'life space' but may be the beginning of a progressive descent into a spiral of reduced mobility. In such patients, encouragement of mobility, assessment for walking or other aids, and a review of the domestic circumstances and need for social support services will require input from remedial therapists and social workers. A home visit by an occupational therapist to look for potential sources of dangers, such as unguarded fires, may be helpful. Where fits are frequent, especially when there is a warning aura, a personal alarm may be useful.

Support

Contact numbers for local branches of the British Epilepsy Association may be useful, though older patients may find the rest of the membership rather young. Spouses, relatives, neighbours and other carers should be advised as to how to manage seizures if they occur.

Drug treatment

Some questions relating to drug treatment:

- When should AEDs be started?
- Which AED should be prescribed?
- How should the dose be adjusted for older people?
- What is the role of AED monitoring?
- What is the prognosis for control?
- Can AEDs be withdrawn?

When should AEDs be started?

Epilepsy is defined as a tendency to recurring seizures, and treatment with AEDs presupposes that a patient does have such a tendency. A single seizure – especially if it has an obvious precipitating cause such as fever or alcohol – does not count as epilepsy, the assumption being that it does not imply an underlying tendency to recurrence. Here the correct approach is not AEDs but removal of the cause.

Where there is a single apparently unprovoked seizure, the decision whether or not to treat with AEDs is more difficult. It will be influenced by several considerations:

- The severity of the index seizure
- The clinician's view as to the likelihood of recurrence (estimates range from 27–80%[48,49])
- The estimate of the risks (such as injury) associated with a recurrent seizure
- The estimated hazards of AEDs
- The credibility given to the notion that 'fits breed fits' i.e. early treatment may prevent epilepsy becoming chronic or intractable

At present, there is inadequate information upon which to base rational decisions as to whether a single unprovoked major seizure in an older person should be treated. Age itself is not a consistent predictor of recurrence although the presence of a clear-cut aetiological factor, such as a focal cerebral lesion, is. The relative dangers of non-treatment (injury resulting from recurrence) and treatment (adverse effects of medication) have never been assessed in a systematic population-based, prospective manner. Until this has been done – and the results of the long-term outcome of trials such as the First[50,51] and MESS[52] studies are available – the decision whether or not to treat a single unprovoked fit partly comes down to personal judgement.[53]

At present, it seems reasonable to treat a single unprovoked major seizure only if it is prolonged or if it has a clear-cut underlying cause such as a previous stroke or a cerebral tumour. Where there is no such cause, and the fit has not been prolonged, the decision is more difficult. In the case of a short-duration generalized convulsive seizure or a partial or non-convulsive seizure, it is probably best to wait. In a patient who has had a single fit it is important to emphasize the need for prompt treatment in future of conditions such as chest infections that might lead to hypoxia and so precipitate further fits. Two or more unprovoked major seizures warrant AED treatment because at this point the risk of recurrence is about 70% in the general adult population[32] and it will probably be higher in the older adult population, where there is more often a continuing underlying cause.

Which AED should be prescribed?

Monotherapy versus combined drug therapy

The majority of adult patients with either primary or secondary generalized seizures or partial seizures can be controlled with a single drug.[54] Nearly 70% of patients can expect a 5-year remission. Phenytoin, carbamazepine and sodium valproate are equally effective as first-line, broad spectrum AEDs.[54] In younger subjects, where monotherapy is unsuccessful, this is very often due to poor compliance or is sometimes associated with a serious underlying cerebral condition. Adding a second drug frequently contributes only additional side-effects. It has been shown that, in patients who are taking more than one drug, withdrawal of the second or third drug may actually improve control. The idea that epilepsy is better controlled with smaller doses of more than one drug makes even less sense in older people who may already be on other medication. If monotherapy with one anti-convulsant gives unsatisfactory control, it is worthwhile trying monotherapy with another.[55] Although monotherapy should be the aim, there will be a proportion of patients who require treatment with two AEDs.

Efficacy trials

Few trials have recruited enough elderly people to be able to compare the efficacy and side-effect profiles of different drugs in this age group. The little information available suggests that no single drug has an overall advantage over any other. In a recent multi-centre comparative trial of efficacy in over 150 patients,[56] both sodium valproate and phenytoin were found to be useful broad spectrum first-line AEDs in elderly-onset seizures. Although there was marginally better seizure control and fewer side-effects with sodium valproate compared to phenytoin, the differences were not statistically significant. Interestingly, actuarial analysis suggested that 78% of patients on valproate and 76% of patients on phenytoin would have a 6-month remission by 12-month follow up – very similar to the findings from monotherapy studies in the general adult population.[54]

At present, then, the evidence suggests that the first-line broad spectrum AEDs – phenytoin, carbamazepine and sodium valproate – have approximately equal efficacy in both generalized tonic-clonic and in partial seizures. The choice of drug will therefore be influenced by considerations of toxicity and, to a lesser extent, cost. The toxicity of AEDs has been investigated extensively, although relatively few studies have included significant numbers of elderly patients.

Side-effects

AEDs may cause acute dose-related, acute idiosyncratic and chronic toxic effects. These adverse effects are usefully summarized in Appleton et al[32] and the reader is strongly advised to be familiar with them when an AED is prescribed.

Neurological side-effects

Gross neurological side-effects include:

- Ataxia
- Dysarthria
- Nystagmus
- Dizziness
- Unsteadiness
- Blurring and doubling of vision
- Reversible dyskinesias
- Asterixis

Reviews of the literature indicate that, although some toxic effects may occur more frequently with certain drugs, there is so much overlap that most neurological side-effects cannot be regarded as specific to any one drug.[54] The effects are generally dose-related and in the general adult population can usually be avoided or minimized by careful dosage titration.

Impact on cognitive function

Effects on cognitive function are of particular relevance. Earlier studies suggested that, of the commonly-used broad spectrum

AEDs, maximum adverse impact was seen with phenytoin and lesser effects with sodium valproate and carbamazepine.[57] Interestingly, a recent detailed study comparing the impact of sodium valproate and phenytoin on various aspects of cognitive function in elderly people, including attention, concentration, psychomotor speed and memory, found little difference between the two drugs[58]. Indeed, phenytoin seemed to have slightly *less* adverse impact on cognitive function than sodium valproate, and neither drug had a major adverse impact. This failure to show a major difference between the two drugs is in keeping with more recent literature comparing the effects of anti-convulsants on cognitive function in the general adult population.[59] Craig and Tallis[58] concluded that, if the dose of AEDs is kept low, adverse cognitive effects are probably not important; and where there are no gross adverse effects, subtle ones are not seen either. Other neurological or neuropsychiatric side-effects may, however, still be significant and there may be important differences in their frequency and severity. This still needs to be systematically studied in patients with elderly-onset seizures.

Non-neurological side-effects

Of the many non-neurological side-effects, osteomalacia[60,61] may be especially relevant, as this is more likely to occur in patients whose poor dietary intake of vitamin D and reduced exposure to sunlight already puts them at risk. Phenytoin in particular induces metabolizing enzymes in the liver and so accelerates metabolism of vitamin D; there may be a case for routine vitamin supplementation in patients on this AED. Sodium valproate, unlike phenytoin or carbamazepine, does not cause hypocalcaemia or reduced vitamin D levels. Carbamazepine-induced hyponatraemia increases significantly with age[62] and may occur at very low doses. The risk of hyponatraemia may be even greater with oxcarbazepine.[63] This will be an important consideration in patients who are on diuretics – especially potassium sparing ones – or who have cardiac failure.

Other considerations

Other considerations may influence the choice of anti-convulsants. Unlike conventional formulation sodium valproate and carbamazepine, phenytoin may be taken in a single daily dose[64] – an advantage in those patients who depend on others to help with their medication. Sustained release valproate which may be taken once a day is now available. Phenytoin also has the advantage that there is a predictable relationship between blood levels and efficacy and between blood levels and side-effects, although physicians should be aware of the implications for dosage increments of the saturation kinetics it exhibits in the therapeutic range (Figure 8). *Dosage adjustments should be in small increments – as little as 25 mg – to prevent a swing from subtherapeutic to toxic blood levels.*

New AEDs

The multi-centre comparative study of AEDs in elderly-onset seizures mentioned earlier[56] indicated a high rate of adverse effects (20%). It might be anticipated that 'minor' adverse effects in older patients, who may be near to the threshold of failure, might translate into a significant difference of function. Herein lies the potential importance of the new generation of AEDs. Two of these look promising for elderly patients: gabapentin because of its simple pharmacokinetics, its efficacy, its comparatively good side-effect profile and its lack of interactions with other drugs;[65] and lamotrigine, because of its simple dosage regime, its efficacy and its comparatively good side-effect profile.[66] Both these drugs have proved effective as adjunctive treatment in patients with partial seizures and secondarily generalized tonic-clonic seizures that could not be satisfactorily controlled with first-line AEDs. Studies are being undertaken to investigate their potential as first-line monotherapy in newly diagnosed cases of epilepsy in elderly patients. At present, they should be used only in patients with seizures that are unresponsive to conventional therapy and hence on the advice of a specialist. If they are to be used as first-line monotherapy in older patients, this should be in the context of an established drug trial at present. More generally, it is impor-

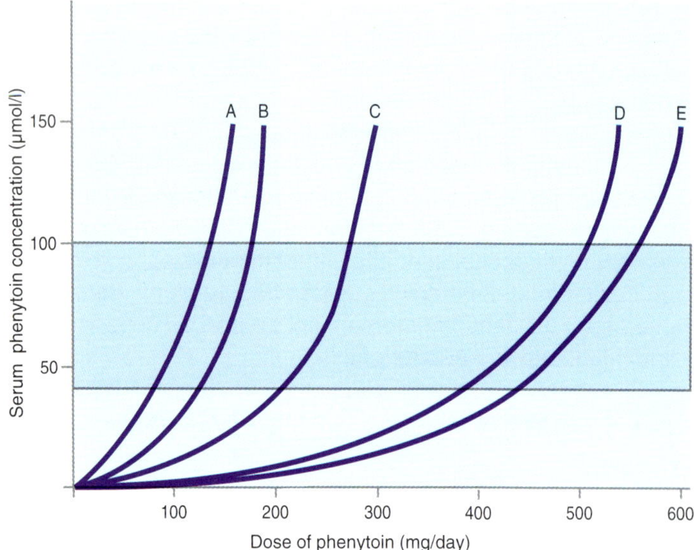

Figure 8

Relationship between blood levels and oral dosage of phenytoin in five patients (A–E) whose steady-state concentrations were measured at several different doses. The coloured area indicates the 'therapeutic range' of serum levels, but is more generous than the usually quoted 40–80 μmol/l (reproduced with kind permission from Laidlaw J, Richens A, Chadwick D. Textbook of Epilepsy, 4th edn. Edinburgh: Churchill Livingstone, 1992).

tant that when the efficacy of drugs has been demonstrated in the younger adult population, they should be evaluated separately in older people; until these studies have been done, such drugs should not be automatically recommended for people with elderly-onset seizures.

Conclusion

For the present, a sensible strategy is for the doctor to use a drug with which he or she is familiar, unless the considerations set out above dictate the choice of another AED. If this works, well and good; if, despite adequate dosage and good compliance, there is poor control, one of the other first-line broad spectrum AEDs should be tried. In a small minority of patients it may be necessary to use more than one AED at a time; such patients should be referred to a physician with a special interest in seizures.

Some patients may not be fully controlled with AEDs. This should not prompt ever-increasing, toxic doses of multiple drugs but a more modest goal. The aim should be to achieve a reduction in fit frequency to tolerable levels without unacceptable side-effects. Feeling continually wretched from the adverse effects of AEDs may be even worse than suffering the intermittent unpleasantness of a fit.

How should the dose be adjusted for older people?

The aphorism that every prescription is an experiment has particular application to older patients in whom the relationship between the oral dose and blood levels is less predictable. Various factors may influence the availability of drugs and consequently the relationship between prescribed dose and serum levels:[67]

- Age-related changes in drug handling
- Concurrent diseases influencing drug handling
- Concurrent medication: drug interactions
- Special compliance problems

Drug handling factors[67]

Plasma protein binding may be reduced, as albumin concentrations tend to be lower in the elderly, especially those that are ill, resulting in higher free concentrations of certain drugs, in particular phenytoin, benzodiazepines and sodium valproate. Single-dose studies have shown reduced clearance of sodium valproate, and in multiple-dose studies the maximum rate of phenytoin elimination and the clearance of unbound valproate were both reduced. The volume of distribution for lipid soluble drugs is increased, probably because of the increase in fatty tissue as a proportion of the total body mass. Taken in conjunction with the reduced clearance, this leads to increased plasma half-time. This particularly applies to phenytoin but not to sodium valproate where, even in the elderly, the half-time is only 11–17 hours.

Our knowledge of age-related pharmacokinetic changes relevant to AEDs is incomplete; moreover, these changes are often derived by comparing mean values for young and old groups and differences *within* these groups may be at least as important as differences *between* them. *To reiterate, age is more important as a source of unpredictable variability than of predictable change.*

Doctors should be aware that generic substitution may be associated with alteration in control and/or an increase in the level of side-effects. This is particularly important with phenytoin, where different preparations have markedly different bioavailability.

Concurrent diseases and medication

Concurrent diseases most likely to be relevant are those affecting metabolism or those which, for a variety of reasons, lead to a further reduction of albumin and hence protein binding. Liver clearance is not flow dependent, so that cardiac failure – except in a terminal, advanced state – should not interfere with metabolism. Renal impairment – which is very common in older patients – is also a less important consideration with the conventional first-line drugs. The multiple pathology associated with old age will inevitably mean multiple medication; many drugs taken by older people interact with AEDs and the latter, of course, interact with one another.

Compliance problems

Patients of all ages comply poorly with AEDs – this is not surprising in view of the chronicity of the treatment, the purely prophylactic nature of the benefit and the frequency of side-effects. There is little evidence, however, that elderly patients are any worse in this respect;[68] nevertheless, poor or variable compliance will be another reason for the lack of a predictable relationship between the prescribed dose and plasma levels.

For all these reasons, it is inappropriate to suggest definite dosage regimes applicable to all elderly patients. *The following general principle should be adhered to: except in cases of emergency, treatment should start at the bottom of the recommended range and the dose should be tailored to the needs of the individual patient.* The initial dose of phenytoin in an elderly person should not be more than 200 mg, possibly lower. Most patients will be controlled on 200–250 mg daily. It would seem reasonable to commence carbamazepine at 100–200 mg total daily dose with a maintenance dose of about 0.6–1.2g daily. Sodium valproate should be started at 400 mg increasing to 1–2 g total daily maintenance dose. Except where fits are frequent and control is a matter of urgency, dosage increases should be gradual. This is particularly applicable to phenytoin where, as already noted, due to saturation kinetics near the therapeutic range, an increment of as little as 25 mg may cause a marked rise in blood levels.

What is the role of AED monitoring?

There is a strong case for judicious drug monitoring, so long as it is appreciated that the most important aspect of *patient* monitoring is not measurement of anti-convulsant levels but information derived from the history and examination. The patient or a relative should keep a record of seizures and, when attending a doctor, the patient should always be accompanied by a well-informed relative, neighbour or carer to ensure that an accurate as possible account of events is obtained. It is important to monitor compliance and make it as easy as possible,[69] by:

- Simplifying regimes
- Giving clear instructions, both orally and written
- Making sure that the medication is clearly labelled
- Making sure that the medication is accessible (child-proof bottles and blister packs may defeat the patient)
- Co-opting the help of carers, relatives and others where appropriate
- Using compliance aids, such as dosette containers
- Having a non-adversarial approach to compliance
- Trying to determine the reason for non-compliance if it is detected

Increasing the dose of AEDs because poor control has been misinterpreted as implying insufficient dosage, when it is in fact due to variable compliance, may lead to disaster. It is important to emphasize the need to take medicine consistently and indefinitely; some elderly patients may have the impression that AEDs only need to be taken when fits occur or as a 'course'.

Underlying the case for drug monitoring is the idea of a **therapeutic range** – a range of plasma or serum levels below which the drug is ineffective and above which it is liable to be toxic. Where there is a narrow therapeutic range and where the relationship between the oral dose and blood levels is unpredictable, there is a strong case for monitoring. Criteria for monitoring have been suggested by Laidlaw et al.[70] Ideally, the clinically effective range should be defined clearly in relation to plasma levels; under such circumstances, measurement of levels in an individual patient would be meaningful and clinically valuable.

The value of anti-convulsant monitoring – in particular its influence on therapeutic decisions – has been demonstrated in several studies of people in all age groups with epilepsy. Lascelles et al[71] showed that 55% of patients had blood levels of anti-convulsants that lay outside the therapeutic range. Reynolds et al[72] found that, of 20% of patients whose epilepsy was not controlled by phenytoin monotherapy, the vast majority of those who did not have extensive brain damage had blood levels outside the normal range. Finally, a more recent survey of an epilepsy clinic found that in nearly one-fifth of visits, a change in management resulted from information about drug concentrations.[73]

AED monitoring may help the recognition of adverse effects of AEDs. These may be subtle and either missed or ascribed to 'old age' or to the worsening of other medical problems. For example, the adverse neuropsychiatric effects of AEDs may be passed off as being due to the effects of cerebrovascular disease. There are more subtle and complex sources of confusion, as when, for example, worsening of cardiac failure due to carbamazepine is attributed to progression of ischaemic heart disease rather than to the effect of the drug. The difficulty of disentangling the adverse effects of AEDs from those of other medication is exacerbated in the biologically aged patient, in whom adverse drug effects may present non-specifically. For example, both digoxin toxicity and AED toxicity may cause increasing mental confusion and in both cases patients may present with increased dependency and the other 'giants of geriatric medicine' – falls, immobility and incontinence.

Knowing AED levels is most useful if it is necessary to answer particular questions or to resolve a particular uncertainty. As it seems reasonable to begin treatment with a lower dose in an elderly patient and as it is also reasonable to aim initially for the lower half of the therapeutic range, it may be appropriate to measure levels routinely once a new patient is established on a particular dose of medication. Furthermore, as the effects of dosage changes are as unpredictable as the effects of the initial dosage, it is important to repeat measurements after a dose alteration prompted by such a measurement.

Therapeutic ranges have been defined for certain populations and there is no certainty that they apply to all populations. As may be expected, the ranges were not established in elderly patients, even less in the type of elderly patients that geriatricians are likely to encounter. It might be possible that toxicity could well occur at levels that fall within the sub-toxic ranges as determined on younger subjects. Doses should not, therefore, be adjusted in fit-free non-toxic patients simply to bring the levels into the 'therapeutic range'. It must be remembered that laboratory results may be incorrect for all sorts of technical reasons, ranging from the time the specimen was taken, through the labelling of the specimen, to the methodology used in the measurement. Indiscriminate and uncritical anti-convulsant monitoring represents a wasted resource.

It is possible that there is no definite lower limit to the therapeutic range. Whether elderly patients in remission can be maintained on lower, even 'sub-therapeutic' doses of AEDs, is something that needs clarifying.[74] It is certainly worthwhile exploring, and should give pause for thought to a physician who, finding an elderly patient on 100 mg of phenytoin daily, concludes that this patient does not require AEDs and abruptly withdraws them. The result may be disastrous.

The value of anti-convulsant monitoring for individual drugs

Phenytoin

Phenytoin is an especially appropriate drug for monitoring:

- Its saturation kinetics mean that there is a non-linear relationship between dose and serum concentration; near the therapeutic range a small adjustment in dose may cause a steep rise in drug level
- In excessive doses, it may produce adverse neuropsychiatric effects which may present non-specifically or be lost in the noise of other neurological and non-neurological pathology
- Variations in kinetics between individuals is more marked than with the other two broad spectrum anti-convulsants
- There is a close correlation, at least at the population level, between blood levels and efficacy, and blood levels and side-effects
- Because of the long half-life of phenytoin, single samples taken randomly give a good approximation of the steady state level

Carbamazepine and sodium valproate

The place of anti-convulsant monitoring is less well-defined in the case of the other two first-line, broad spectrum anti-convulsants. Single random samples will not necessarily reflect steady-state levels because of their shorter half-lives. Moreover, the relationship between serum concentrations and control is less clear cut than with phenytoin. There does, however, appear to be a definite, although smaller, role for monitoring carbamazepine and sodium valproate.

Therapeutic monitoring of carbamazepine has been usefully reviewed by Brodie and Hallworth.[75] They point out that the dosage of carbamazepine is a poor predictor of serum concentration (although, after the initial period of enzyme induction, the relationship between dose and plasma concentration in an individual is relatively linear) and that many of the side-effects do appear to be concentration dependent. The relationship between serum carbamazepine concentration and clinical response is, however, complicated by variable metabolism to its active metabolite and individual pharmacodynamic variability. The values given for the therapeutic range should be interpreted with caution: seizure control may be achieved throughout a very wide range of concentrations – from below 4 mg/l to above 16 mg/l. Moreover, a single measurement may be meaningless because of great variations of concentration during a dosage interval. Both peak (3–4 hours after a dose) and trough (at the time of the next dose) levels should be measured. Despite these reservations, it would seem to be reasonable to use therapeutic monitoring of carbamazepine where there is uncertainty about toxic effects, where control is poor and where compliance is uncertain.

The place of monitoring sodium valproate levels is even more uncertain and the concept of a therapeutic range for this drug even less precise.[76] Certain side-effects, such as tremor, appear to be concentration dependent.[77] There is, however, little correlation between valproate concentration and its pharmacological effect[78] and there may be diurnal variation in drug clearance and repeated levels on the same dose may show wide variation. Peak levels occur at 1–4 hours after ingestion.[79] A patient requiring a consistently high concentration should probably be changed to a different anti-convulsant. Monitoring may help to rationalize treatment in patients on polypharmacy (valproate increases the circulating levels of other anti-convulsants, while other enzyme-inducing anti-convulsants reduce valproate levels), and identify the cause for treatment failure when a patient is on an apparently adequate dose. Samples should be taken at a standard time in relation to doses.

When interpreting the results of plasma drug concentrations, it must be remembered that in the elderly a greater proportion of the drug will be in the free state[67] – due mainly, though not entirely, to lower albumin concentrations. Drug concentrations in the cerebrospinal fluid will tend to approximate the free concentration in the plasma; the same total plasma concentrations will probably therefore indicate a higher brain concentration than in a younger patient. This age effect is small with phenytoin but larger with valproate.

What is the prognosis?

Control of fits

There is little information on the proportion of elderly-onset epilepsy patients who are satisfactorily controlled with AEDs. A retrospective study[80] of admissions to a geriatric unit found that re-admission due to poor control was very uncommon. In a recent comparison of phenytoin with sodium valproate,[56] failure due to poor control was found in only 2% of patients on sodium valproate and 4% of subjects on phenytoin (this difference was not significant), although in 10% and 14% of cases, respectively, treatment was withdrawn due to adverse effects. A recent report from the National General Practice Study of Epilepsy found that 9 years after the index seizure, 68% of subjects with definite epilepsy had had a 5-year remission and that age was not relevant.[81]

Mortality

Mortality is increased in epileptic patients. However, the relative increase – the standard mortality ratio – may be less marked in those diagnosed over 60 years of age than in those diagnosed in youth or middle age. Hauser et al[82] found that the death rate from cardiac disease was increased in patients with elderly-onset epilepsy but that the incidence of sudden cardiac death was increased only in patients with symptomatic epilepsy, in whom cerebrovascular disease was the probable cause. Luhdorf et al[83] followed 251 patients for a minimum period of 2 years. The survival rate at 6 years was 60% of the expected rate (i.e. the rate in the general population). Most deaths were due to cerebrovascular disease or tumours and, when patients with overt symptoms due to this were excluded, mortality was no higher than that of the age-matched population. It would appear that epilepsy *per se* does not increase mortality.

In summary, what little evidence is available suggests that, in the absence of significant progressive disease, the prognosis both for control of seizures and for survival is good in elderly-onset cases.

Can AEDs be withdrawn?

When should AEDs be withdrawn in patients with elderly-onset seizures? The literature (for example, the Medical Research Council AED withdrawal study[84]) addresses much younger populations. Late onset epilepsy, partial and secondarily generalized seizures (which are of course more common in the elderly) and the presence of known cerebral pathology (also more common in elderly epileptic patients) are, however, associated with an increased rate of relapse, and the conclusion may have to be reluctantly reached that withdrawal of therapy should not be attempted in most elderly patients who were given anti-convulsants for a good reason in the first place.

Epilepsy clinics and epilepsy services

There are few specialist services for older people with epilepsy. Elderly people with seizures may fall between two stools – specialist geriatrics services and specialist epilepsy services. Whether this amounts to an argument for specialist geriatric epilepsy services is not clear. If such services were developed, specialist diagnostic facilities would need to be a crucial element because the most difficult phase in management is confirming the diagnosis of seizures.

The particular needs of elderly patients with seizures may perhaps be best served by a geriatrician with an interest in and enthusiasm for seizures. He or she might be better offering a service for the management of 'funny turns'. Diagnosis-specific clinics – such as epilepsy clinics and syncope clinics – tend to pre-judge diagnoses. Enthusiasts for the former may have a bias towards the diagnosis of epilepsy and for the latter towards syncope: we tend to find what we seek.

The clinic should be supported by, and reach out to, the wider geriatric medical services and community services. There should be clear definition of the roles of general practitioners and specialists in what will, inevitably in a chronic disease, be 'shared care'.

Areas for research

For the reasons given at the begining of this book, geriatric epileptology is a relatively under-developed and under-researched field. Areas ripe for research include:

- Causes of seizures
- The physical impact of seizures: injuries
- The psychosocial impact of seizures
- When to use AEDs
- The role of the new generation of AEDs
- The organization of epilepsy services

Causes of seizures

Although it now seems clear that cerebrovascular disease is the commonest cause of seizures in old age, the connection may be exaggerated because of the near-universality of CT scan evidence of vascular disease in old people. More studies are needed to determine the frequency and type of cerebral tumours as a cause.

The physical impact of seizures

Seizures might be expected to have more adverse physical effects in elderly people. Research is required to determine whether this is the case – for example, how frequently fractures occur in association with epilepsy.

The psychosocial impact of seizures

Jacoby and colleagues[85] have emphasized how the

"impact of a chronic illness is experienced not only through its physical symptoms, but also as a result of its effect on psychosocial functioning. In the case of an illness such as epilepsy, where the physical manifestations are transient, the psychosocial consequences may, with time, come to be of greater concern."

We know little or nothing about this in older people. What do they think about seizures? What misconceptions and fears do they have and how much do these contribute to increased dependency and shrinking life-space? It is necessary to determine the information needs of older people and how these can best be met.

When to use anti-convulsants

Should a single unprovoked tonic-clonic seizure be treated in old age or should treatment be delayed until two or more seizures have occurred? What are the chances of recurrence where there is no overt cause? Prospective studies are needed to answer related questions, such as how easily seizures can be controlled in old age, and whether epilepsy in elderly people can be controlled with lower blood levels of anti-convulsants than are necessary in younger people.

The role of the newer generation of anti-epileptic drugs

What is the place of monotherapy using the new generation of anti-convulsants in the *de novo* treatment of elderly onset seizures? Studies addressing this question should focus not simply on the traditional end-points such as seizure control, as the importance of newer AEDs may lie more in reducing subtle adverse effects on gait and mobility than in improving seizure control, especially as 'minor' effects of this sort may, in a frail elderly person, translate into significant dysfunction.

The organization of epilepsy services

How best can a service for elderly people with seizures be provided? What are the elements of an optimal overall comprehensive service? Who should provide such a service and how should it be evaluated?

If answers to these questions were available, the management of seizures in old age would be considerably better than it is now.

Appendix – Driving and epilepsy: New regulations for ordinary licence holders – August 1994

- A patient may drive only if he or she is free of epileptic attacks during the year before the date when the licence is granted

or

- If epileptic attacks occur only during sleep, the patient must have had a sleep-only pattern for 3 years or more

and

- His or her driving must be unlikely to endanger the public where driving is compromised by drug treatment or associated neurological or neuropsychiatric disturbances.

Single seizures – not regarded as epilepsy by the DVLA unless a continuing liability can be shown (usually by EEG or imaging). However, the DVLA usually prohibits driving for 12 months after a single seizure.

Provoked seizures – precipitated by exceptional non-recurring circumstances in non-epileptic subjects. Driving is usually allowed once the provoking factor has been successfully treated or removed. The precipitating factor must be truly exceptional. Alcohol and illicit drugs do not qualify.

Mild seizures – e.g. myoclonic jerks and seizures not associated with loss of conciousness. These are treated the same as other attacks.

Attacks occurring during changes in drug treatment – regulations apply. Licence will be barred regardless of whether deliberate or accidental.
Driving should be suspended during changes in drug treatment (advisory not regulatory).
When drugs are being totally withdrawn, driving should be suspended from the time withdrawal begins until 6 months after completion.

EEG changes – without overt seizures, these are not usually a bar to driving. The exception is unequivocal 3 Hz spike/wave in primary generalized seizures.

From: Shorvon S. Epilepsy and driving. *BMJ* 1995; **310**: 885–6.
Advice for doctors about driving and epilepsy is available from the medical adviser, Driving and Vehicle Licensing Agency, Swansea SA99 1TU (telephone 01792 783686).

References

1. Craig I, Tallis RC. General practitioner knowledge and management of elderly-onset epilepsy. *Care of the Elderly* 1991;**3**:69–72.
2. Godfrey JW, Roberts MA, Caird FI. Epilpetic seizures in the elderly: 2 diagnostic problems. *Age Ageing* 1982;**11**:29–34.
3. Godfrey JW. Misleading presentation of epilepsy in elderly people. *Age Ageing* 1989;**18**:17–20.
4. Downton JH. *Falls in the Elderly* (London: Edward Arnold, 1993).
5. Sander JWAS, Hart YM, Johnson AL, Shorvon SD. National General Practice Study of Epilepsy: newly diagnosed epileptic seizures in general population. *Lancet* 1990;**336**:1267–70.
6. Chadwick D. Epilepsy after first seizures: risks and implications. *J Neurol Neurosurg Psychiatry* 1991;**54**:385–7.
7. Beghi E, Ciccione A, and The First Seizure Trial Group. Recurrence after a first unprovoked seizure. Is it still a controversial issue? *Seizure* 1992;**2**:5–10.
8. Commission on Classification and Terminology of the International League Against Epilepsy. Proposal for revised clinical and electroencephalographic classification of epileptic seizures. *Epilepsia* 1981;**22**:489–501.
9. Commission on Classification and Terminology of the International League Against Epilepsy. Proposal for revised classification of epilepsies and epileptic syndromes. *Epilepsia* 1989;**30**:389–99.
10. Hauser WA, Kurland LT. The epidemiology of epilepsy in Rochester, Minnesota, 1935 through 1967. *Epilepsia* 1975;**16**:1–66.
11. Hauser WA, Annegers JF, Kurland LT. Prevalence of epilepsy in Rochester, Minnesota: 1940–1980. *Epilepsia* 1991;**32**:429–45.
12. Hauser WA, Annegers JF, Kurland LT. Incidence of epilepsy and unprovoked seizures in Rochester, Minnesota: 1935–1984. *Epilepsia* 1993;**34**:453–68.
13. Luhdorf K, Jensen LK, Plesner AM. Epilepsy in the elderly: incidence, social function, and disability. *Epilepsia* 1986;**27**:135–41.
14. Tallis RC, Craig I, Hall G, Dean A. How common are epileptic seizures in old age? *Age Ageing* 1991;**20**:442–8.
15. Loiseau J, Loiseau P, Duche B, Guyot M, Dartigues J-F, Aublot B. A survey of epileptic disorders in Southwest France: seizures in elderly patients. *Ann Neurol* 1990;**27**:232–7.
16. Luhdorf K, Jensen LK, Plesner A. Etiology of seizures in the elderly. *Epilepsia* 1986;**27**:458–63.

17. Sung C-Y, Chu N-S. Epileptic seizures in elderly people: aetiology and seizure type. *Age Ageing* 1990;**19**:25–30.
18. Kilpatrick CJ, Davis SM, Tress BM, Rossitor SC, Hopper JL, Vandendriesen ML. Epileptic seizures in acute stroke. *Arch Neurol* 1990;**47**:157–60.
19. Lancman ME, Golimstok A, Norscini J, Granillo R. Risk factors for developing seizures after stroke. *Epilepsia* 1993;**34**:141–3.
20. Shorvon SD, Gilliatt RW, Cox TCS, Yu YL. Evidence of vascular disease from CT scanning in late onset epilepsy. *J Neurol Neurosurg Psychiatry* 1984;**47**:225–30.
21. Shinton RA, Gill JS, Melnick SC, Gupta AK, Beevers DG. The frequency, characteristics and prognosis of epileptic seizures at the onset of stroke. *J Neurol Neurosurg Psychiatry* 1988;**51**:273–6.
22. Mcareavey BJ, Ballinger BR, Fenton GW. Epileptic seizures in elderly patients with dementia. *Epilepsia* 1992;**33**:657–60.
23. Heckmatt JA. Seizure induction by alcohol in patients with epilepsy. Experience in two hospitals. *J R Soc Med* 1990;**83**:6–9.
24. Lechtenberg R, Worner TM. Total ethanol consumption as a seizure risk factor in alcoholics. *Acta Neurol Scand* 1992;**85**:90–4.
25. Tallis RC. Biological ageing, illness in old age, and geriatric medicine. *J Hong Kong Geriatrics Soc* 1993;**4(1)**:4–11.
26. Chadwick DW. Convulsions associated with drug therapy. *Adverse Drug Reaction Bulletin* 1981;**87**:316–19.
27. Swift C. Drug-induced neurological disease. In: Tallis R, ed. *The Clinical Neurology of Old Age* (Chichester: John Wiley and Sons, 1988): 391–406.
28. Puxtey J. The neurological complications of metabolic nutritional and endocrine disorders. In: Tallis R, ed. *The Clinical Neurology of Old Age* (Chichester: John Wiley and Sons, 1988): 309–22.
29. Hankey GJ. Cerebrovascular disease: a clinical approach. *Rev Clin Gerontology* 1994;**4**:289–310.
30. Jarvik LF, Lavretsky EP, Neshkes RE. Dementia and delirium in old age. In: Brocklehurst JC, Tallis RC, Fillit HM, eds. *Textbook of Geriatric Medicine and Gerontology* (Edinburgh: Churchill Livingstone, 1992): 326–49.
31. Miller JW, Peterson RC, Metter EJ, Milliken CH, Yanagihara T. Transient global amnesia: clinical characteristics and prognosis. *Neurology* 1987;**37**:733–7.
32. Appleton R, Baker G, Chadwick D, Smith D. *Epilepsy*, 3rd edn (London: Martin Dunitz, 1993): 26.
33. McIntosh S, DaCosta D, Kenny RA. Outcome of an integrated approach to the investigation of dizziness, falls and syncope in elderly patients referred to a 'syncope' clinic. *Age Ageing* 1993;**22**:53–8.
34. Schott GD, Macleod AA, Jewitt ED. Cardiac arrhythmias that masquerade as epilepsy. *BMJ* 1977;**i**:1454–7.
35. Grubb BP. Differentiation of convulsive syncope and epilepsy with head-up tilt testing. *Ann Intern Med* 1991;**115**:871–6.
36. Kogeorgos J, Scott DF, Swash M. Epileptic dizziness. *BMJ* 1981;**282**:687–9.
37. Blumer D. Epilepsy and disorders of mood. *Adv Neurol* 1991;**55**:185–95.
38. Rowan AJ. Ictal amnesia and fugue states. *Adv Neurol* 1991;**55**:357–67.
39. Ellis JM, Lee SI. Acute prolonged confusion in later life as an ictal state. *Epilepsia* 1978;**19**:119–28.
40. Jamal GA, Fowler CJ, Leslie K, Prior PF, Gawler J. Non-convulsive status epilepticus as a cause of acute confusional state in the over-60 age group. *J Neurol Neurosurg Psychiatry* 1988;**51**:738.
41. Norris JW, Hachinski VC. Mis-diagnosis of stroke. *Lancet* 1982;**i**:328–31.

42. Fine W. Post hemiplegic epilepsy in the elderly. *BMJ* 1967;**1**:199–201.
43. Smith J. Clinical neurophysiology in the elderly. In: Tallis RC, ed. *The Clinical Neurology of Old Age* (Chichester: John Wiley and Sons, 1989): 89–97.
44. Ramirez-Lassepas M, Cipolle RJ, Morillo LR, Gumnit RJ. Value of computed tomography scan in the evaluation of adult patients after their first seizure. *Ann Neurol* 1984;**15**:436–43.
45. Young AC, Costanzi JB, Mohr PD, Forbes WS. Is routine computerised axial tomography in epilepsy worthwhile? *Lancet* 1982;**ii**:1446–7.
46. Chadwick D. How far to investigate the elderly patient with epilepsy. In: Tallis RC, ed. *Epilepsy and the Elderly* (London: Royal Society of Medicine Services, 1988):21–30.
47. Kilpatrick CJ, Tress BM, O'Donnell C, Rossitor C, Hopper JL. Magnetic resonance imaging and late-onset epilepsy. *Epilepsia* 1991;**32**:358–64.
48. Chadwick D. Epilepsy after first seizures: risks and implications. *J Neurol Neurosurg Psychiatry* 1991;**54**:385–7.
49. Berg AT, Shinnar S. The risk of seizure recurrence following a first unprovoked seizure: a quantitative review. *Neurology* 1991;**41**:965–72.
50. Beghi E, Ciccione A, and The First Seizure Trial Group. Recurrence after a first unprovoked seizure. Is it still a controversial issue? *Seizure* 1992;**2**:5–10.
51. Beghi E, and the First Seizure Trial Group. A randomised clinical trial of the efficacy and safety of the treatment of the first unprovoked epileptic seizure. *Neuroepidemiology* 1992;**11**:50–1.
52. Medical Research Council. *Multi-centre study of early epilepsy and single seizures (MESS).* Ongoing study.
53. Reynolds EH, Chadwick D. Controversies in treatment and management. Do anti-convulsants alter the natural course of epilepsy? *BMJ* 1995;**310**:176–7.
54. Treiman DM. Efficacy and safety of antiepileptic drugs: a review of controlled trials. *Epilepsia* 1987;**28 (suppl 3)**:S1–8.
55. Schmidt D, Richter K. Alternative single anti-convulsant therapy for refractory epilepsy. *Ann Neurol* 1986;**19**:85–7.
56. Tallis RC, Easter D, Craig I. Multicentre trial of sodium valproate and phenytoin in elderly patients with newly diagnosed epilepsy. *Age Ageing* 1994;**23 (suppl 2)**:P5.
57. Trimble MR. Anti-convulsant drugs and cognitive function: a review of the literature. *Epilepsia* 1987;**28 (suppl 3)**:S37–45.
58. Craig I, Tallis R. The impact of sodium valproate and phenytoin on cognitive function in elderly patients: results of a single-blind randomised comparative study. *Epilepsia* 1994;**35**:381–90.
59. Meador KM, Loring DW, Huh K, Gallagher BB, King DW. Comparative congitive effects of anti-convulsants. *Neurology* 1990;**40**:391–4.
60. Ashworth B, Horn DB. Evidence of osteomalacia in an outpatient group of adult epileptics. *Epilepsia* 1977;**18**:37–43.
61. Gough H, Goggin T, Bissessar A, Baker M, Crowley M, Callaghan N. A comparative study of the relative influence of different anti-convulsants, UV exposure and diet on vitamin D and calcium metabolism in out-patients with epilepsy. *Q J Med* 1986;**59**:569–77.
62. Lahr MB. Hyponatraemia during carbamazepine therapy. *Clin Pharmacol Ther* 1985;**37**:693–6.
63. Houtkooper MA, Lammertsma A, Meyer JWA, Oxcarbazepine: a possible alternative to carbamazepine. *Epilepsia* 1987;**28**:693–8.
64. O'Driscoll K, Ghadiali E, Crawford P, Chadwick D. A comparison of single daily dose and divided dose of phenytoin in epileptic outpatients. *Acta Therapeutica* 1985;**11**:375–85.

65. Chadwick D. The role of gabapentin in epilepsy management. In: Chadwick D, ed. *New Trends in Epilepsy Management: the Role of Gabapentin* (London: Royal Society of Medicine Services, 1993):59–65.
66. Richens A. Overview of the clinical efficacy of lamotrigine. *Epilepsia* 1991;**32 (suppl 2)**:S13–16.
67. Mawer G. Specific pharmacokinetic and pharmacodynamic problems of anticonvulsant drugs in the elderly. In: Tallis RC, ed. *Epilepsy and the Elderly* (London: Royal Society of Medicine Services, 1988):21–30.
68. Weintraub M. Compliance in the elderly. *Clin Geriatr Med* **6(2)** (Philadelphia: WB Saunders Co, 1990).
69. Leppik IE. How to get patients with epilepsy to take their medication. The problem of non-compliance. *Postgrad Med* 1990;**88**:253–6.
70. Laidlaw J, Richens A, Oxley J. *A Textbook of Epilepsy* (London: Churchill Livingstone, 1988).
71. Lascelles PT, Kocen RS, Reynolds EH. The distribution of plasma phenytoin levels in epileptic patients. *J Neurol Neurosurg Psychiatry* 1970;**33**:501–9.
72. Reynolds EH, Shorvon SD, Galbraith AW, Chadwick D, Dellaportas CI, Vydelingum L. Phenytoin monotherapy for epilepsy: a long term prospective study, assisted by serum level monitoring, in previously untreated patients. *Epilepsia* 1981;**22**: 475–88.
73. McKee PJW, Larkin JG, Brodie AF, Percy-Robb IW, Brodie MJ. Five years of anti-convulsant monitoring on site at the epilepsy clinic. *Ther Drug Monit* 1993; **15**: 83–90.
74. Callaghan N, Kenny RA, O'Neill B, Crowley M, Goggin T. A prospective study between carbamazepine, phenytoin and sodium valproate as monotherapy in previously untreated and recently diagnosed patients with epilepsy. *J Neurol Neurosurg Psychiatry* 1985;**48**:639–44.
75. Brodie MJ, Hallworth MJ. Therapeutic monitoring of carbamazepine. *Hospital Update* 1987:57–63.
76. Anon. Sodium valproate [editorial]. *Lancet* 1988;**ii**:1229–31.
77. Dreifuss FE, Langer DH. Side-effects of valproate. *Am J Med* 1988;**88 (suppl 1A)**:34–41.
78. Minns RA, Brown JK, Blackwood DHR, McQueen JK. Valproate levels in children with epilepsy. *Lancet* 1982;**i**:677–8.
79. Loiseau P, Cenraud B, Levy RH. Diurnal variations in steady-state plasma concentrations of valproic acid in epileptic patients. *Clin Pharmacokinet* 1982;**7**:544–52.
80. Ghose K. Incidence and presentation of epilepsy in an acute geriatric unit [Abstract]. *Proceedings of the Fourth British, Danish and Dutch Epilepsy Congress, Amsterdam, September 1988:* page 61.
81. Cockerell OC, Johnson AL, Sander JWAS, Hart YM, Shorvon SD. Remission of epilepsy: results from the National General Practice Study of Epilepsy. *Lancet* 1995; **346**: 140–4.
82. Hauser WA, Annegers JF, Elveback LR. Mortality in patients with epilepsy. *Epilepsia* 1980;**21**:399–412.
83. Luhdorf K, Jensen LK, Plessner AM. Epilepsy in the elderly: life expectancy and causes of death. *Acta Neurol Scand* 1978;**76**:183–90.
84. Medical Research Council Antiepileptic Withdrawal Study Group. A randomised study of antiepileptic drug withdrawal in patients in remission of epilepsy. *New Engl J Med* 1991;**337**:1175–80.
85. Jacoby A, Baker G, Smith D, Dewey M, Chadwick D. Measuring the impact of epilepsy: the development of a novel scale. *Epilepsy Research* 1995 (in press).

Index

Page numbers in *italic* refer to the figures